D

56 Smoothie Recipes for Losing Weight, Healthier
Living, Radiant Skin, & Shiny Hair.

Em Davis

Contents

Forward

We all know that we need to eat our fruits and veggies, but it can be difficult to get all of the servings we need in any one day; especially in this fast paced, and busy world. Many people desire to be healthy. They want to lose weight, to detoxify their body, to have more energy, and to feel great. Fruits and vegetables are the best way to achieve that as they have all of the vitamins and nutrients necessary for optimal health.

But don't despair if you find it difficult to eat all of the recommended servings of fruits and vegetables. There is a way to cheat the system. Smoothies. Smoothies are an excellent way to get your fruits and vegetables in an easy to eat and digest way. You make a smoothie in minutes, put in a cup with a lid and straw and take it to go. You can drink it on your way to work while everyone else is drinking coffee. And a smoothie made from fresh produce is better than any late for boosting energy and waking you up. And you don't need any high tech equipment.. All you need is a knife to cut up the fruit or veggies of choice, and a blender. That's it.

You may be thinking, "But I don't have time to make a smoothie before work in the morning." No worries. I usually put all the ingredients together the night before. Then all I have to do is put it in the blender, blend it at high speed for 30 seconds to a minute, pour it in one of those to go cups, which you can get at any store, rinse the blender, and go. When I get home, I get my blender out and mix up another smoothie. It's easy. It's simple. It's fast.

Try the 30 day Smoothie challenge. This means for 30 days eat a smoothie with your breakfast—not instead of your normal breakfast, but with it. For instance, if you usually eat a bagel in the morning, eat that bagel with a smoothie. In the afternoon, or evening, have another smoothie. I eat a spinach salad every night for supper. Now I eat the same salad with a smoothie as my beverage. Remember, smoothies are not to replace the vegetables you are currently eating; they are meant to add to it. Do a smoothie twice a day for 30 days and you will start to notice a difference in how you feel and look. Your hair will look healthier. Your skin will look clearer and more radiant. You'll have more energy and you may even drop a pound or two. Though if you are following your smoothie with a double bacon cheeseburger you can forget about the weight loss.

All of the recipes in this book can be made in 5 minutes and in a blender. So what are you waiting for. Start blending today!

Banana Crème Pie

1 banana

1 cup crème

1 tsp. vanilla

1 tsp. honey

1. Put in blender and blend until smooth. Serve in a glass.

Pumpkin Pie

1 8 oz. can of pumpkin puree

1 cup milk

1 tsp. honey

1/4 tsp. cinnamon

1/4 tsp. ginger

1/8 tsp. nutmeg

1. Put in blender and blend until smooth. Serve in a glass.

Coconut Cream Peach

1/2 cup coconut flakes

1 peach, pitted and peeled

1 cup milk (or use coconut milk)

1. Put in blender and blend until smooth. Serve in a glass.

Kale-icious

2 cups kale

1/2 tsp. lemon juice

1 cup water

1 tsp. honey

1. Put in blender and blend until smooth. Serve in a glass.

Creamed Spinach

2 cups spinach

1/2 cup cream

1/2 cup milk

1 tsp. basil

1. Put in blender and blend until smooth. Serve in a glass.

Pina Colada

1/2 cup coconut flakes

1 8 oz. can of pineapple chunks

1 cup coconut milk

1 tsp. honey

1. Put in blender and blend until smooth. Serve in a glass.

Strawberries and Cream

1 cup strawberries

1 cup cream

1. Put in blender and blend until smooth. Serve in a glass.

Berry-licious

1 12 oz. package of frozen mixed berries

1/4 cup dried Goji berries

1 cup milk

1 tsp. honey

1. Put in blender and blend until smooth. Serve in a glass.

Liver Cleanse

1 cup kale

1 cup spinach

1 cup arugula

1/2 cup fresh cilantro

1/2 cup fresh parsley

1 cup water

2 tsp. honey

1. Put in blender and blend until smooth. Serve in a glass.

Yummy Zucchini

1 small zucchini, cut into chunks

1/2 cup water

1/4 tsp. ginger

1 tsp. honey

1. Put in blender and blend until smooth. Serve in a glass.

Pumpkin Cucumber

1 small cucumber, cut into chunks

1 8 oz. can pumpkin puree

1 cup milk

1 tsp. honey

1/4 tsp. cinnamon

1. Put in blender and blend until smooth. Serve in a glass.

Cucumber Surprise

1 cucumber, cut into chunks

1 cup kale

1/2 cup strawberries

1 cup milk

1. Put in blender and blend until smooth. Serve in a glass.

Pomegranate Margarita

1 cup pomegranate seeds

1 cup strawberries

1/2 a lime

1 cup water

1. Put in blender and blend until smooth. Serve in a glass.

Blueberry World

1 cup blueberries, you can use frozen)

1/2 cup raisins

1 cup milk

1 tsp. honey

1. Put in blender and blend until smooth. Serve in a glass.

Strawberry Kiwi

1 cup strawberries

1 kiwi, peeled and sliced

1/8 tsp. ginger

1 cup milk

1 tsp. honey

1. Put in blender and blend until smooth. Serve in a glass.

Orange Marmalade

1 orange, peeled and sliced

1/2 a lime, peeled

1/2 cup cherries, pitted

1/2 cup water

1 tsp. honey

1. Put in blender and blend until smooth. Serve in a glass.

Sweet and Sour Lemon

2 lemons, peeled

1 lime, peeled

1/2 cup water

3 tsp. honey

1. Put in blender and blend until smooth. Serve in a glass.

Pear-Apple

1 pear, cored and sliced

1 apple, cored and sliced

1/8 tsp. cinnamon

1 cup milk

1. Put in blender and blend until smooth. Serve in a glass.

Celery with Apple Punch

1 apple, cored and sliced

2 stalks celery, cut up

1 cup milk (or try almond milk)

1/4 cup sunflower seeds

1 tsp. honey

1. Put in blender and blend until smooth. Serve in a glass.

Celery Surprise

4 stalks celery, cut up

1/2 cup cherries, pitted

1/2 cup pomegranate seeds

1 cup water

1 tsp. honey

1. Put in blender and blend until smooth. Serve in a glass.

Buttermilk Soufflé

1 egg (if you don't want to eat a raw egg, then cook it before putting it in the blender.)

1 cup buttermilk

1 cup coconut flakes

1 tsp. honey

2 tsp. cinnamon

1 tsp. ginger

1. Put in blender and blend until smooth. Serve in a glass.

Strawberry Banana

1 banana

1 cup strawberries

1 cup water

1. Put in blender and blend until smooth. Serve in a glass.

Banana Peach and Apple

1 banana

1 peach, pitted and sliced

1 cup strawberries

1 cup milk

1. Put in blender and blend until smooth. Serve in a glass.

Tropical Mango

1 8 oz. can pineapple chunks

1 mango, pitted and sliced (or use 1/2 cup dried mango)

1 banana

1/2 cup pitted cherries

1 1/2 cups milk

1 tsp. honey

1. Put in blender and blend until smooth. Serve in a glass.

Pineapple Papaya

1 cup Kale

1 cup papya chunks

1 8 oz. can of pineapple chunks

3 mint leaves

1 cup milk

2 tsp. honey

1. Put in blender and blend until smooth. Serve in a glass.

Coconut Papaya

1 cup coconut flakes

1 cup papaya chunks

1/2 cup kale

1 cup coconut milk

1. Put in blender and blend until smooth. Serve in a glass.

Creamy Papaya with Strawberries

1 cup papaya chunks

1 cup strawberries

1 cup cream

1. Put in blender and blend until smooth. Serve in a glass.

Cranberry Orange

1 orange, peeled

1/2 cup frozen cranberries

1 cup water

3 tsp. honey

1. Put in blender and blend until smooth. Serve in a glass.

Cranberry Apple

1 apple, cored and sliced

1/ cup frozen cranberries

1 cup water

1/2 cup almonds

1 tsp. honey

1. Put in blender and blend until smooth. Serve in a glass.

Grape Vino

1 cup grapes

1/2 blackberries

1/2 cup raspberries

1 cup milk

1. Put in blender and blend until smooth. Serve in a glass.

Garlic Breath

1 cup collard greens

1 clove garlic

1 carrot

1/4 tsp. ground ginger

1. Put in blender and blend until smooth. Serve in a glass.

Green Surprise

1 small cucumber, cut up

1 cup kale

1 kiwi, peeled and sliced

1/4 cup sunflower seeds

1/2 cup water

1 tsp. honey

1. Put in blender and blend until smooth. Serve in a glass.

-

Butternut Berry

1 cup butternut squash chunks

1 cup blueberries

1/4 tsp. cinnamon

1 cup milk

1 tsp. honey

1. Put in blender and blend until smooth. Serve in a glass.

Creamed Broccoli

1 cup broccoli, raw and cut up

1 cup coconut milk

1/2 cup almonds

1 tsp. honey

1. Put in blender and blend until smooth. Serve in a glass.

Almond Berry

1 cup frozen mixed berries.

1/2 cup almonds

1 cup milk

1 tsp. honey

1. Put in blender and blend until smooth. Serve in a glass.

Creamed Cauliflower

1 cup cauliflower, raw and cut up

1 cup coconut milk

1 /2 cup sunflower seeds

1/2 cup raisins

1 tsp. honey

1. Put in blender and blend until smooth. Serve in a glass.

Sweet Potato Almond

1 small sweet potato, cut up into small chunks

1/2 cup almonds

1 cup milk

1/2 tsp. cinnamon

1. Put in blender and blend until smooth. Serve in a glass.

Kale Cauliflower Carrot

1 cup kale

2 carrots, peeled and cut up

1/3 cup cauliflower florets

1/2 cup dates, pitted

1 cup water

1. Put in blender and blend until smooth. Serve in a glass.

Carrot Apple

1 apple, cored and sliced

3 carrots, peeled and cut up

1 cup water

1 tsp. lemon juice

1. Put in blender and blend until smooth. Serve in a glass.

Peachy Pears

1 peach, pitted and sliced

1 pear, cored and sliced

1 cup spinach

1 cup milk

1. Put in blender and blend until smooth. Serve in a glass.

Spinach Pear

1 pear, cored and sliced

1 cup spinach

1/2 cup pumpkin seeds

1 cup milk

1. Put in blender and blend until smooth. Serve in a glass.

Pineapple Melon

1 8 oz. can pineapple chunks

1 banana

1 cup watermelon chunks

1/2 cup water

1. Put in blender and blend until smooth. Serve in a glass.

Honey Nut

1 cup Honeydew chunks

1/2 cup almonds

1 cup cantaloupe chunks

1/2 cup water

1. Put in blender and blend until smooth. Serve in a glass.

Watermelon Green

1 cup watermelon chunks

1 cup spinach

1 cup kale

1 cup water

1. Put in blender and blend until smooth. Serve in a glass.

Cantaloupe Banana

1 banana

1 cup cantaloupe chunks

1 cup milk

1/2 cup almonds

1. Put in blender and blend until smooth. Serve in a glass.

Pomegranate Melon

1 cup spinach

1 cup pomegranate seeds

1 cup cantaloupe chunks

1 cup coconut milk

1. Put in blender and blend until smooth. Serve in a glass.

Casaba Berry

1 cup frozen mixed berries

1 cup casaba chunks

1/2 cup kale

1 cup almond milk

1. Put in blender and blend until smooth. Serve in a glass.

Herblicious

1 cup spinach

3 sage leaves

1/2 cup fresh cilantro

1/2 cup fresh parsley

1/2 cup fresh rosemary

1 cup water

1 tsp. honey

1. Put in blender and blend until smooth. Serve in a glass.

Hawaiian Hula

1 banana

1 8 oz. can of pineapple chunks

1 cup spinach

1 cup coconut flakes

1 cup milk

1. Put in blender and blend until smooth. Serve in a glass.

Coconut Cantaloupe

1 cup coconut flakes

1 cup cantaloupe chunks

1/4 cup sunflower seeds

1 cup coconut milk

1. Put in blender and blend until smooth. Serve in a glass.

Rosemary Thyme

1 cup spinach

1 cup arugula

1/4 cup fresh rosemary

1/8 cup fresh thyme

1 cup coconut milk

1/2 cup almonds

1. Put in blender and blend until smooth. Serve in a glass.

Plum Nectar

1 plums, sliced

1 peach, sliced

1 cup spinach

1 cup milk

1. Put in blender and blend until smooth. Serve in a glass.

Plum Berry

2 plums, sliced

1 cup strawberries

1 cup raspberries

1/2 cup coconut flakes

1 cup milk

1. Put in blender and blend until smooth. Serve in a glass.

Squashed Greens

1 small yellow squash, sliced

1 cup kale

1 cup spinach

1 cup coconut flakes

1 cup water

1. Put in blender and blend until smooth. Serve in a glass.

Eggplant Berry

1 small eggplant, cut up into chunks(Use half of it if it's too big.)

1 cup strawberries

1/2 cup blueberries

1 cup milk (Use almond milk for a different flavor.)

1. Put in blender and blend until smooth. Serve in a glass.

Minty Chocolate Mouse

4 oz. chocolate (Use 75 % cacao or higher.)

3 mint leaves

1 cup spinach

1/2 cup almond

3 tsp. honey

1 cup half and half (or use cream to make it really creamy.)

1. Put in blender and blend until smooth. Serve in a glass.

More by Em Davis

Why buy jam when you can make your own?

Get Em Davis' 35 Delectable Jams: All Sugar Free and Breadmaker Friendly

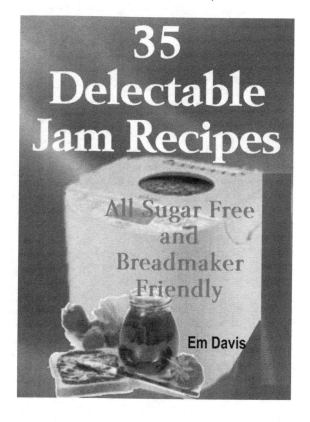

Don't forget the benefits of cooking

with stevia

Stevia: 55 Naturally Sweetened Recipes

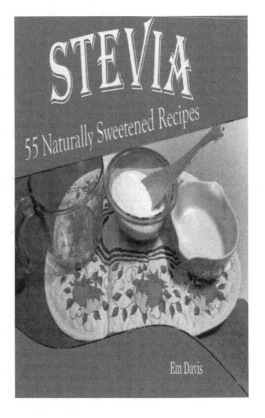

Detox For Life 2

57 More Smoothie Recipes for Losing Weight, Healthier Living, Radiant Skin, & Shiny Hair.

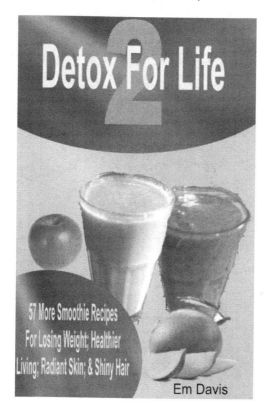

Afterward

I want to thank you for purchasing this recipe book. I hope you make good use of it and enjoy the benefits of eating healthy without sacrificing taste. Please consider leaving a review. Reviews are very helpful for others. You can even mention some of your favorite recipes and make your own smoothie combinations.

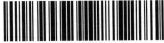

Made in the USA
San Bernardino, CA
21 April 2015